Alzheimer's

Based on a true story...
24/7 with Ms. Adele

by

Yvonne D. Knight

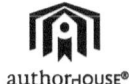

authorHOUSE®

AuthorHouse™
1663 Liberty Drive, Suite 200
Bloomington, IN 47403
www.authorhouse.com
Phone: 1-800-839-8640

First published by AuthorHouse   8/29/2007

ISBN: 978-1-4343-2996-7 (sc)

Library of Congress Control Number: 2007905628

Printed in the United States of America
Bloomington, Indiana

This book is printed on acid-free paper.

This story is dedicated to Alzheimer sufferers all over the world, their families and the caregivers who supply them with the love and care they so desperately need. I also wish to take this opportunity to thank God for the inspiration to put these ten years into words for others to experience.

About Adele

Adele was born, Adele Seeman May 30, 1911 in Detroit, Michigan, the last of four children. Her parents were Jewish immigrants. She attended school in the Detroit public school system and upon graduation, went on to college. After graduating from college, Adele returned to become a teacher in the same Detroit public school system where she began her education.

Teaching became her passion. She was blessed with a teaching career of 43 years.

In 1939, she was introduced to Peter Fergal, who was to become her husband. They married in the same year and were able to enjoy each others company for nearly 30 years. Adele, now in her late fifties, lost Peter to a heart attack. She was now alone except for relatives, for she and Peter never had children.

Adele continued to teach school after Peters passing until she retired in her late sixties. After her retirement, she spent much of her time reading. In addition, she would often visit nursing homes in the area and read to the patients. It was through these cumulative visits that Adele had become adamant she would never want to spend one day in a nursing home.

Finally, when Adele was in her early to mid 80's, she moved from her private home to an independent living facility for seniors.

She continued her reading and began to spend more time alone. As she approached here late 80's, she began to realize her mental capacity was diminishing.

Entr, Yvnn!

About Yvonne

Yvonne, a first generation American, is the third daughter from a family of six children. She was born to an Italian mother and a French Canadian father. She was raised in a loving environment in the Berkshire Hills of Massachusetts. Yvonne attended Catholic schools in Pittsfield, Massachusetts, her birthplace. She dropped out of High school to get married at sixteen years old. She and her husband Philip had six premature children. Yvonne lavished love on her children and was an excellent mother. Her husband suffered from mental illness and Yvonne's early years of family life were a struggle to raise her six children. She often depended on Welfare and Commodities to survive. Later in life, she worked for fifteen years as a caregiver for the elderly in care homes. She also worked in an office for five years. Her husband, Philip who she was married to for 32 years, committed suicide in 1992. At this time her empty nest and her nurturing nature allowed her to be open to Adele and Adele recognized her as a perfect caregiver.

About the Story

This true story is based on the progression of Alzheimer's disease in a lady named Adele. Adele is presently 95 years old. She retired after forty two years of school teaching. Widowed in her late fifties and without children, Adele is the last of her three siblings: two sisters and one brother. She is alone in her illness except for a few nieces and nephews.

Adele met Yvonne in 1997 when Adele was eighty six year's old and when Alzheimer's was first diagnosed. Yvonne agreed to be her caregiver and wanted to make a difference in her life.

The story will cover the nine years that Yvonne cared for Adele-up until the present. Adele changed Yvonne and taught her many things on this journey they have shared. Some may find the humor, others will see tragedy as the two of them deal daily with this devastating disease.

Yvonne learned to love tiny Adele as a daughter would love her mother facing the same illness. This story is

Yvonne's way of telling the world her personal experience with Alzheimer's and her relationship with the precious human being, Adele.

Contents

Stage I

My journey with Adele began in 1997 while I was in the process of looking for work. Because I had fifteen years experience working in nursing homes, I decided to apply at an independent senior housing complex as a concierge. I got the position and started working in January of the same year. I enjoyed working around the elderly, as I had in the past. Days passed uneventfully as I became friendly with many of the residents of the complex.

One evening I was conducting our normal systematic door checks. Door checks involved making sure that the residents had his/her door card turned to the 'good night' all is well side. When I got to the fourth floor apartment # 402, the card was still on 'good day'. Not a good sign! I knocked on the door to be sure the resident was ok.

The resident, Ms. Adele, opened her door in a frantic frenzy. I had apparently awakened her and she appeared to be frightened. I will never forget how cute she looked. She stood only 4'9". A bit of a lady, in her flannel night gown with ruffled wrists and hem was a sight that brought a smile to my face.

She had been having a bad dream, I believe. She kept saying: "My niece Allene was in a car accident and she had blood all over her face." I spent some time calming her down and assuring her everything was alright. Finally she was composed enough to excuse herself to use the bathroom. I felt she was ok enough to finish my door checks; however, I made a mental note to recheck 'Adele' before my shift was over. This night began the start of our long and caring friendship.

I was surprised to find that the very next day when I arrived at work Ms. Adele was waiting for me at the concierge desk to talk. She knew my shift started at 3pm and she would be there everyday thereafter to visit and chat with me. Some days I would drive her to the bank to conduct business, as a favor, on my lunch hour. We became close friends. A strong, natural bond began to weave us together.

Adele began to tell me her life story. She was a school teacher for forty -two years. I learned that she is Jewish, a widow, and that her husband Peter died when she was fifty-eight years old. She and Peter never had children. She told me she had a brother, Abe, who had passed away years ago. She spoke of her sisters: May and Jenny. She talked more about Jenny, probably because Jenny had recently passed away.

Adele has several nieces and nephews. Her niece Allene seemed to be the one she spoke of the most. Adele recently heard that this niece had been diagnosed with jaw cancer. I suddenly connected my initial meeting with Adele. Adele was dreaming about this niece being in a car accident because she had just heard about the diagnosis of cancer. Adele was preoccupied with concern over her favorite niece that she loved so much.

I believe Adele was already in Stage I of Alzheimer's. She was not processing information correctly. It had been very recent that she-on her own- had sold her car. She made the decision to sell the car and to stop driving. She said she did not feel safe driving anymore. I believe Adele was intelligent enough to recognize the first signs of this disease in her own person!

Days turned into weeks.

On reporting in to work daily we were given an update on residents. On this one particular day I was told that my little friend Adele had caused an uproar at 2am that morning. She had been hanging over the 4th floor railing yelling: "My mother is dead, my mother is dead." This unusual behavior was unacceptable in this senior complex. Her niece Allene was called in to handle the situation and get Adele the help she needed.

Very soon thereafter I received a phone call from Allene wanting to discuss Adele's recent behavior. Allene also informed me that Adele had been diagnosed with Alzheimer's. Adele was now forgetting to take her medications. After a doctor's visit, the family had decided to have Adele attend Alzheimer's classes three times a week.

Allene asked me during that phone conversation if I would consider being Adele's personal caregiver during the day. I was to make sure she was taken care of and that she took her medications. I agreed and started personal care of Adele in March 1997.

Everyday thereafter I would go to her apartment in the morning. I made sure she had breakfast, helped her wash and dress, and gave her medications on time. I would take her to and from her Alzheimer's classes. If she did not have classes we went shopping or stayed in to do little things around her apartment that she may need help with. For dinner, Adele would attend group meals at the senior home. I became more involved with her illness as she started calling me in the wee hours of the morning. Adele would awaken occasionally between 2am and 4am very frightened. She would call me and I would calm her down and reassure her I would be seeing her in a couple of hours.

After a few months of caring for Adele, she began to share her biggest fears with me. She shared that she feared going into a nursing home. One day she asked if I would stay with her until she died so she would not die in a nursing home. I promised her that if I was well enough to care for her I would indeed stay with her. I did tell her that her family would be the deciding factor on her care. She was quieted like a child on hearing that I would never leave her and felt sure her family would respect her wishes also.

She was so delighted with the prospect of being cared for by someone who loved her that she wanted us to go on a cruise to celebrate. In late July 1997 we checked with different travel agencies. We both agreed to take a fall cruise into Canada. It was to be twelve days long on the Crystal Cruise ship. We left for the cruise September 1997.

The idea of going on this expensive cruise was probably the most exciting event of my life. Adele had paid almost $10,000.00 for the two of us. My imagination of what a luxurious vacation meant and traveling for two weeks with an Alzheimer's patient were not one and the same dream. Alzheimer's does not make fun dreams of day to day living but a cruise with an Alzheimer's patient can be classified as a nightmare or bad comedy at least.

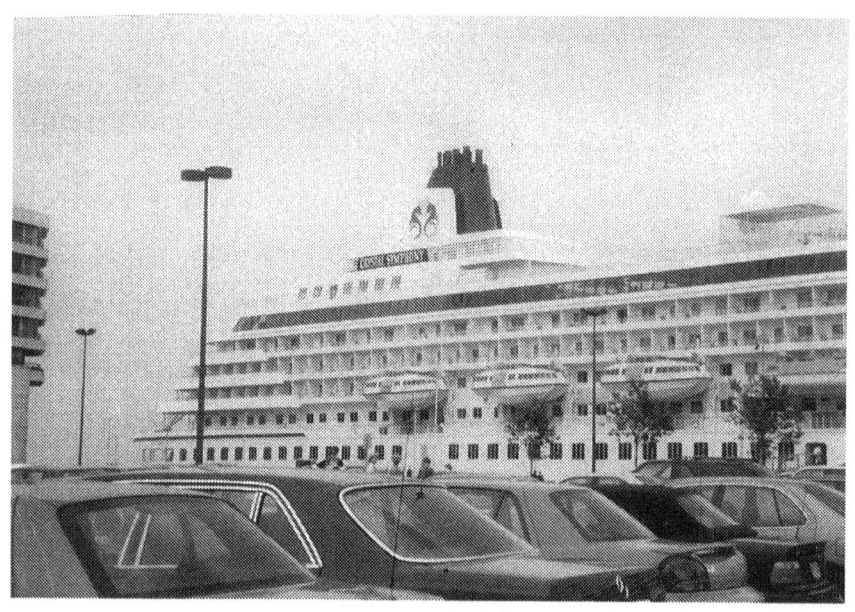

Crystal Cruise Ship 1997

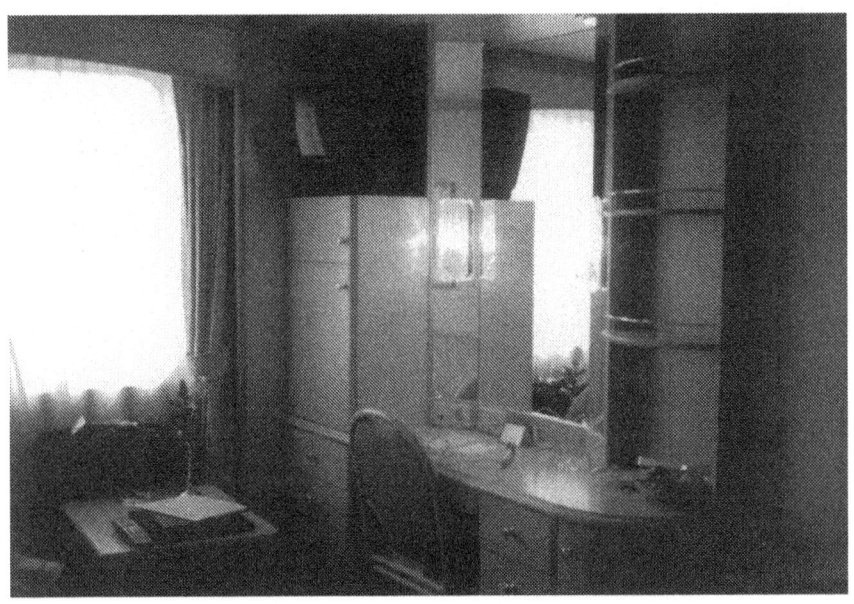

Cruise Cabin 1997

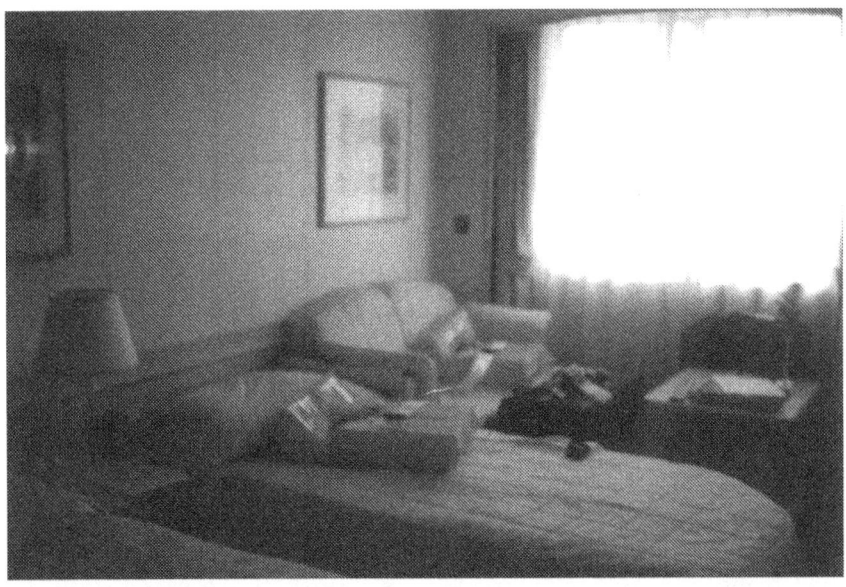

The Cruise/Nightmare/Bad Comedy

The cruise package limousine arrived at the senior home to pick us up and whisk us to the airport. Upon arriving in Montreal, Canada the tour bus took us to the Crystal cruise ship. The tour bus driver announced the different buildings of interest to the passengers. All of a sudden Ms. Adele bursts out: "Oh, he thinks he's so smart, why doesn't he shut up?" I tried to quite her down all the while feeling pretty embarrassed myself for both of us. As we left the bus I tried to explain to the bus driver that Adele had an illness. He said it was alright but I feel sure he did not understand. I apologized. Except for this outburst all went pretty smooth this first leg of the journey with Ms. Adele.

We arrived at the ship and were escorted to our cabin room. I began unpacking the bags when the captain announced over the loud speakers that all passengers were to put on their life jackets and report on deck in fifteen minutes for an emergency trial run. Great, Captain! Adele announces she needs to use the bathroom-big emergency= for real! She had already gone potty in her pants-too late-so its clean-up time in the tiny on board cabin. Finally we are all cleaned up causing us to be a little late for the emergency trial run on deck. By this time I am laughing so hard, just thinking, if these people knew what had just taken place with Adele and I minutes earlier, and now, here we are standing here with these crazy looking orange life jackets on as if nothing has ever happened.

Things did not get much better as the day progressed. Day one of my dream vacation was turning into: 'my life with an Alzheimer's patient who is a dear friend'.

For dinner, Adele and I attended an Italian restaurant aboard ship. After we had been seated for around fifteen minutes Adele was convinced we were being ignored and proceeded to yell loudly: "Give us some service, we paid for this cruise". For the rest of the cruise I had our meals brought to the cabin to avoid another incident. I knew she could not help herself because of the Alzheimer's, but the embarrassment was just too much for me.

I was confident that after taking her medications Adele would settle down and relax and the vacation would be semi-normal. This was not to be. For some strange reason the medications did not work on this cruise and I was never able to leave Adele alone for one moment on the entire trip.

The first night on board ship I looked over the activities that we could attend. The movie theatre sounded like an ok idea until the next day at a movie Ms. Adele started snoring so loud we had to leave the theatre. She did not sleep at night so movies put her to sleep: fast and loud!

All in all, dream vacation turned into a 'ready to go home soon' trip. I do not recommend a cruise vacation for Alzheimer's patients and their caregivers. In fact, I was so glad to get home and just spend eight hours a day on duty and then go to my own home to totally relax.

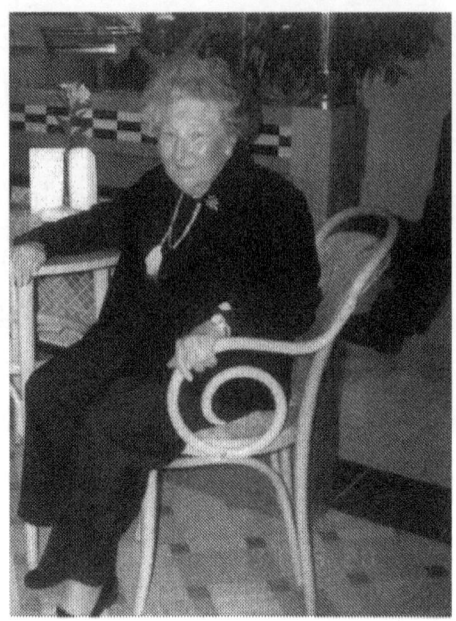

Adele at Cruise Ship coffee shop

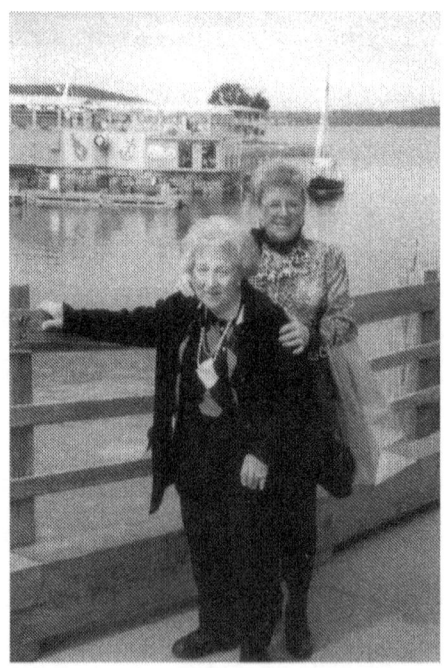

Adele & Yvonne – Cruise 1997

Back at the senior home

Never a dull moment with Adele as days and months passed at the senior home. Usually on Sundays after church services I went by to check on Adele. On this particular day I opened her apartment door to an overpowering stench of feces. I walked down her hallway to the bathroom to find all the white towels smeared with brown mess. Adele strolls out from her TV sitting room unaware of a problem. I ask her: "Adele, do you know there is bowel movement all over the bathroom?" She answers: "Oh, stop making mountains out of mole hills". I had to laugh so I would not cry. I went into her TV room where she had taken feces and thrown them all over the place. With my high heels and church garb on I chose to laugh it off, roll up my sleeves and clean up the mess. It was part of the job and the disease.

As the days and weeks passed Adele got very argumentative. At other times, she would cry for no apparent reason. Something as simple as writing a check for an electric bill was unmanageable. There were times she looked at me and had no clue as to who I was.

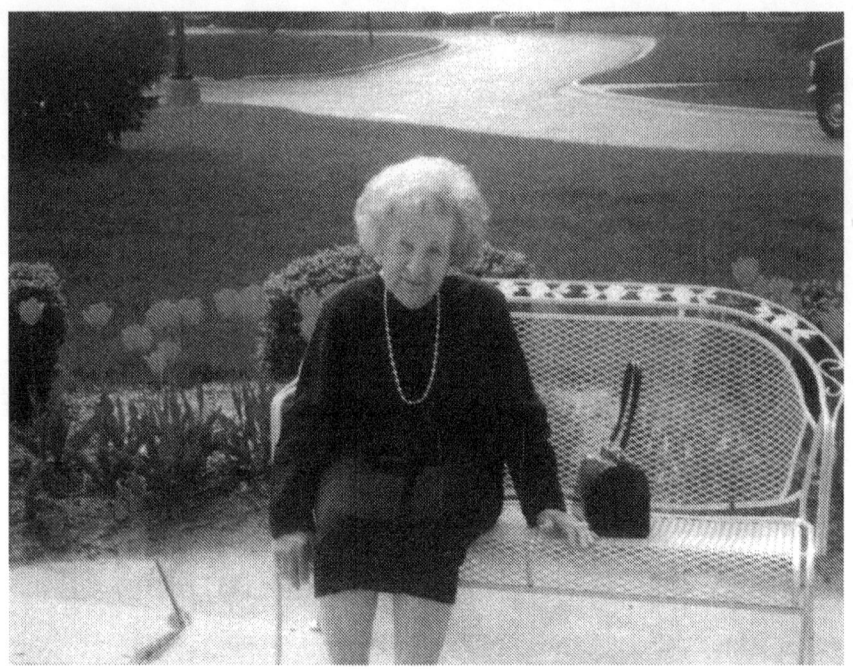

Adele outside of Senior Home 1997

One morning I arrived at Adele's apartment. She was all excited telling me she had made breakfast for me. She brought me into her little sitting room. She had set up a card table with half of her real silverware, elegant glasses and dishes with nothing in them. She had sugar and milk only, on this breakfast treat for me. The gesture warmed my heart for this lovely woman.

On one other occasion I arrived at her apartment where her nine foot tall bookcase was emptied on the floor. She had been an avid reader early on, so there were many books. When I questioned her about what might have happened she replied that they just fell. I did not question her anymore on this one.

Once she requested that she be moved from the fourth floor to the second floor. I asked her why she would want to move. She replied that when she decided to jump she would not have far to fall. I laughed but after a few moments realized that she was serious about wanting to die.

In early 1997 I arrived early at Adele's to take her shopping for nightgowns before her doctor appointment. She was a little agitated because she did not want to spend any money. We bought the needed nightgowns and were off to her doctor's appointment.

After arriving at the doctor's office, I went around to help Adele out of the car. We walked arm in arm up the sidewalk towards the office. Adele's foot either caught in the concrete or she had momentarily forgotten how to walk but she ended up falling face first to the ground before I could catch her.

I called out to a passing stranger to get help for us. Her doctor came out of the office and immediately called an ambulance. I followed the ambulance in my car to the hospital to be with Adele.

By the time she had been placed into a room her entire face was black and blue. She had a broken nose and various bumps and bruises. She was released when the doctors were comfortably sure she was ok, but from my point of view she was never quite the same. I called her niece, Allene, who was in Florida at the time. I told Allene about Adele's fall. I also told her that I did not feel comfortable leaving Adele alone at night. I stayed with Adele until Allene arrived back into town. After Allene visited Adele, she also, agreed that all was not well with her aunt and the fall had mysteriously caused her Alzheimer's disease to progress.

Adele began talking much less and her hands started to curl into fists. This made holding a fork or spoon impossible. Stage I had drawn to a close to bring on Stage II and begin my life of 24X7 with Adele.

It was at this point that I decided to start keeping notes of my experiences with Adele. My little Adele does not communicate any longer and I miss that. Occasionally, I read to her because she was such a lover of books and to help pass the time.

The bond had been formed between us. I had already learned a life time of wisdom from this lady. I prayed to the Lord for her, and that I would retain the strength to care for her. I prayed deeply for all the people, victims, caregivers and families of victims of this dreaded disease. I prayed for a cure.

Stage II

By 1998 I was living full time at Adele's apartment. I went to my home once a day to get mail and do our laundry. Adele went everywhere with me. I was with her and she with me 24x7.

After her fall she was more passive but she still could get into mischief. Like a child, if I did not watch her every second, chaos could result. She could be sitting quietly in a chair and the next moment, be out the door.

On one occasion, while I was in the kitchen preparing a snack for the both of us, she walked out of the apartment got on an elevator and would get off randomly on one of the seven floors in the building. She kept me running from floor to floor as she got into and out of the elevators. Unexpected events progressed as the disease continued to progress.

Because I am a heavy sleeper, early morning wakefulness became a real problem with my little charge, Adele. On several occasions, in the wee hours of the dawn (say 2am or

3am) she striped off her nightgown for a stroll through the complex. Another resident would see her parading in the nude and call security. Security would then call me and bring Adele back to her apartment wrapped in his or her jacket.

This was a source of embarrassment so I called her niece. Allene called the doctor to schedule Adele for a new workup. Adele was admitted to the hospital for one week to run tests. I went to her side everyday for as long as the hospital allowed. The tests showed little, and all the doctors could conclude was that Adele was in another stage of Alzheimer's. My new challenge was simply to keep her from getting out at night while I was asleep.

I decided to put my mattress on the floor in front of the door of her apartment to eliminate the nightly strolls in the buff. In order to get out now, she would have to step on me and this would surely wake me up. This was a success! Many nights thereafter she would wake me up. She would be ready to stroll in her birthday suit. I would put her little gown back on and tuck her into bed once again.

One night, Adele went to use the bathroom alone during the night. Unknown to me she had wet all over the bathroom floor. I got up myself to use the bathroom after her mishap and with only the night light on I did not see the puddle on the bath room floor. I fell flat on my back as I slid over the urine in my bare feet. I ran my big toe into the sink cabinet. I thought out loud: "Dear Lord, I've broken my toe for sure!!!" It was not broken but it sure hurt for some time.

You may be really laughing right now, as I am, but at the time it happened, rest assured, I was not laughing. The months passed without time to dwell on sorrow. Being constantly present is vital in the care of an Alzheimer's patient.

In early 1998 Adele and I went out somewhere everyday. We liked garage sales and on one occasion I got a really good price on an item. When we got back into the car I made the careless remark that I had 'jewed' the person down. To my surprise Adele took note of the comment and reprimanded me saying: "That is not a nice way to talk, Yvonne" thoughtlessly, I had forgotten that Adele is Jewish. I apologized to her and told her I was sorry, but thought how odd that with her disease she was so alert at times.

There were times when Adele could really be a 'cut-up' comic on purpose. One day, upon returning to the apartment, another resident asked me why Adele walks hunched over. I tried to be polite in the face of this rudeness, so I answered, Adele has arthritis in her back. When we got inside the apartment, I voiced my displeasure out loud: "Why doesn't that busybody go jump in a river?" I ended up in a roaring laugh when Adele answered me: "Yeah and two lakes, too!!"

Niece Allene had now assumed all of Adele's financial affairs. In the past Allene would take Adele to the opera or out to lunch on the week-ends but now we did not see much of Allene. Allene and I would talk on the phone regarding Adele's welfare and other matters of interest.

Allene and her husband Marty started to travel quite frequently. Because of her illness, I assumed she wanted more time with her husband. I suspected she was worse than she told us but I never wanted to upset Adele, so much was not said on this topic.

Walking became more difficult for Adele so we obtained a wheelchair to make getting around easier on both of us. She did continue to walk some but very slowly. She even had problems sitting up in the chair without falling out. We remedied that problem by obtaining a wheelchair seatbelt and buckling her in. She objected at first but I convinced her it was for her own safety, like in a car.

Every Sunday we went to church together and the wheelchair made that much easier. She liked church even though it was Christian and she was raised Jewish. On one occasion, while I was ironing and listening to a Christian TV program, I heard Adele saying the sinner's prayer to accept the Lord Jesus into her heart. This brought tears to my eyes as I thought: "Yes, Jesus was Jewish also like this sweet lady".

In the fall of 1998 my youngest son was getting married and another son was turning thirty. They decided to join the celebrations together. Adele and I flew to New Jersey from Detroit, Michigan to attend the Wedding/Birthday parties. Medication and the wheelchair made this trip much easier than the cruise. Stage II is fast becoming Stage III in my friend's disease. I still read occasionally to her, though she understands little.

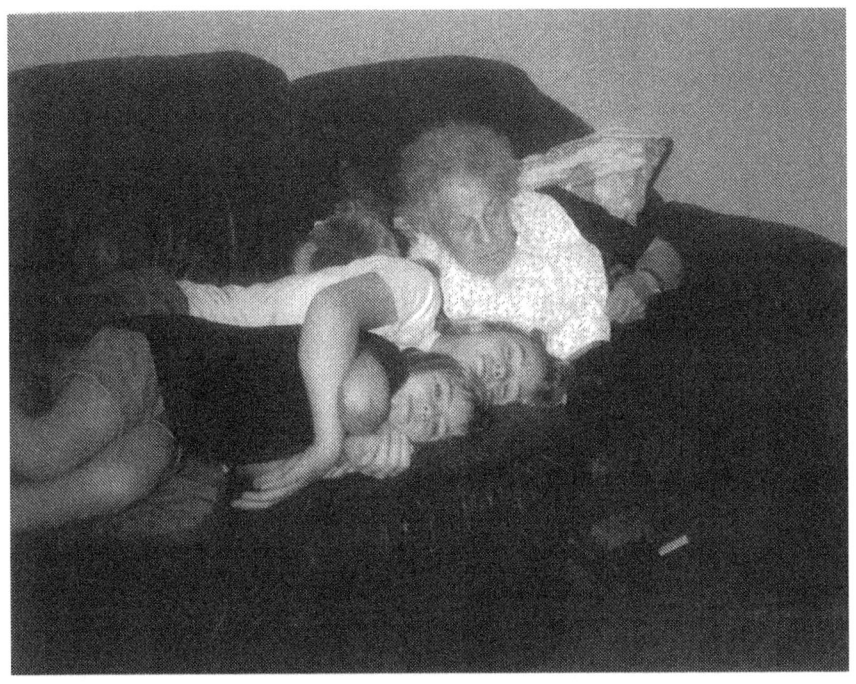

Adele, with Yvonne's 2 grand children, Katie & Kaley
New Jersey 1998

*As the disease goes on, symptoms are more easily noticed and become serious enough to cause people with Alzheimer's disease or their family members to seek medical help. For example, people in the later stages of Alzheimer's disease may forget how to do simple tasks, like brushing their teeth or combing their hair. They can no longer think clearly.

*They begin to have problems speaking, understanding, reading, or writing. Later on, people with Alzheimer's disease may become anxious or aggressive, or wander away from home. Eventually, patients need total care.

Stage III

In 1999 we got a hospital bed for Adele. She is not capable of getting up during the night because she is not steady on her feet and falling could be fatal. I now sleep in the same room with her. In the night she often calls out for her sister Jenny, her husband Peter, and her brother Abe (all deceased). She calls out for her niece Allene also.

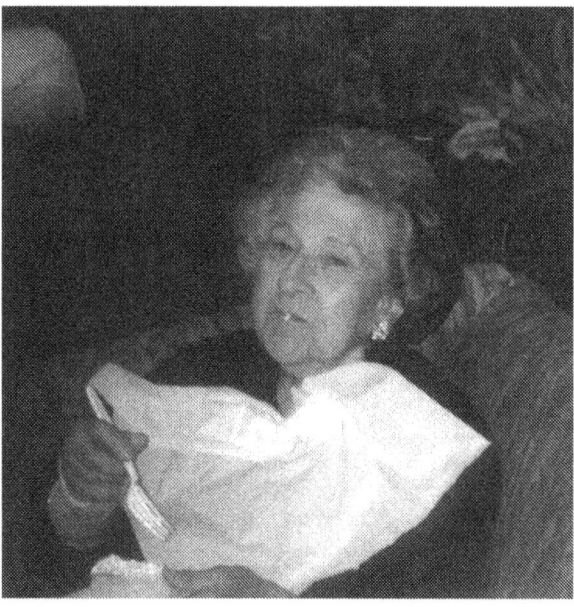

Adele's 88th Birthday party at Allenes' home 1999

On May 30th of this year Adele turned 88. She shared the same birthday with her niece Allene and this year Allene invited her to her home for a birthday party with other family members.

By July of 1999 Allene was in and out of the hospital for cancer treatments. On September 28th, I got the call that Allene had died. This was indeed a sad day. Allene was a lovely lady. I dreaded to tell Adele. I gave Adele a shower, sat her in her wheel chair and sat down in front of her. I reminded her of how sick Allene had been. She agreed with me so I proceeded to tell her of the death. Adele eyes filled and spilled like faucets. She understood and in a moment we were clutching each other in comfort both of us crying like babies at our loss. Such a beautiful person and how we loved that lady.

This death had yet another profound effect on my friend Adele. She stopped calling out names of family members. It was almost as if she had willingly lost all memory. This saddened me to see another low for my friend.

Marty, Allene's husband, took over the finances for Adele.

In late fall 1999; I planned for Adele and I to attend my granddaughter's December wedding in Indiana. I went to the mall to pick up a dress ordered for the occasion. It was late Sunday afternoon after church and Adele had fallen asleep on the way. Instead of disturbing her I parked the car in the handicapped section and ran in to pick up the dress. I was not gone over ten minutes when I heard sirens on the way out. I arrived at my car to find a fire ambulance, a regular ambulance, two police cars, a fire truck, and security all surrounding my car and Adele. My heart stopped as I thought something had happened to Adele. When I got closer I saw Adele talking to the police officer.

After talking to the police officer myself, I learned that Adele had awakened, undid her seat belt, got out of the car and proceeded to tell passerby's that she was lost. When I explained the situation to the police they advised me not to leave her unattended for even one second.

No one had to worry about that mistake happening again. From that day on asleep or awake, no matter the inconvenience, I pulled the wheelchair out of the trunk and took Ms. Adele

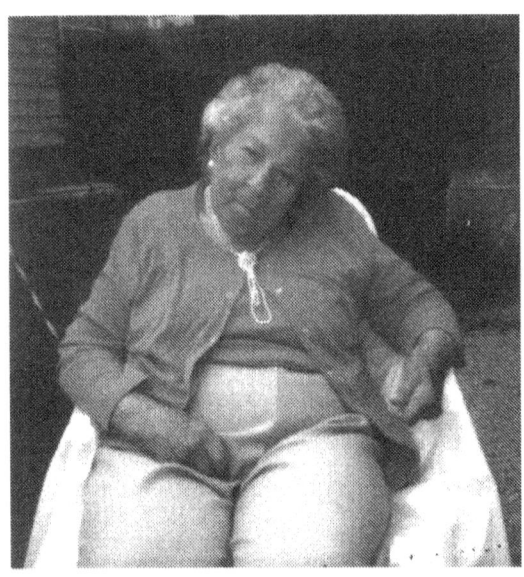

Adele's 89 Birthday

with me everywhere.

Stage III is ending with my friend becoming more and more like a toddler or infant, from a mental aspect. I continue to sit by the little one's bed and read to her. She smiles.

Stage IV

In the year 2000 -the millennium- life with Adele had become very quiet. I started to notice that she had stopped eating much. It was almost as if she forgot how to chew food even though she has all her own teeth.

On my own, I started to puree her food in a food chopper. She began to eat better. She became unable to swallow her medication any longer. I thus began to crush and mix them with applesauce.

By summer of this year, I was taking Adele to my home almost everyday as I gardened outside as she watched. She got a nice little tan and seemed to enjoy the sunlight. I was still taking her to church with me and to the mall and garage sales.

I wanted to start attending Bible study and this was the year I did. This did not last too long, however, because the time from 9:30am to noon was too long for Adele. The first time she had a bowel movement in her *Depends*, I dropped the class and we just went to regular services. Adele is 89 year's old and I am happy to have her in my life.

Adele was placed on a daily dose of an anti-biotic for urinary track infections around this time by her urologist. At this time I had been caring for Adele in this progressive disease for over three years. Her regular doctor informed me and her family that I had put an extension on her life by my care of her. This warmed my heart.

Many of the resident's of this care home envied the fact that Adele was able to go somewhere everyday of the week with me. I believe many of the residents' lives could have been extended by more outside activities. Many of her friends at the complex died, while she continued on walking a little and going out daily, snow, rain, or shine. Her walking tapered down more and more until Stage V set in.

Stage V

By 2001 Adele had to wear *Depend* diapers all the time because she no longer had control of her urine or waste. Instead of oatmeal I bought baby cereal as she could not handle the texture of regular oatmeal to swallow.

It was this year that I learned that Marty had been diagnosed with Lou Gehrigs' disease. I knew this was not a good thing and I did not tell Adele at this time. She really did not understand much by this time. She did not even remember who Marty was. I saw less and less of Marty. His secretary was my contact. Marty started to travel and he had good and bad days with the disease.

In May Adele turned 90 years old. We celebrated in Indiana where my daughter had given birth at the time.

Adele and I continue the visits to the dentist and doctor appointments and our usual outings for most of this year. One of those usual days was September 11th. I was thinking of all the pointless deaths of young people and people in the

Yvonne D. Knight

prime of life that took place on that terrible day. I glanced over at Adele and prayed: "Lord God, help me to understand the meaning of life".

That year ended with Adele and I spending the Holidays at home alone but very content and quiet.

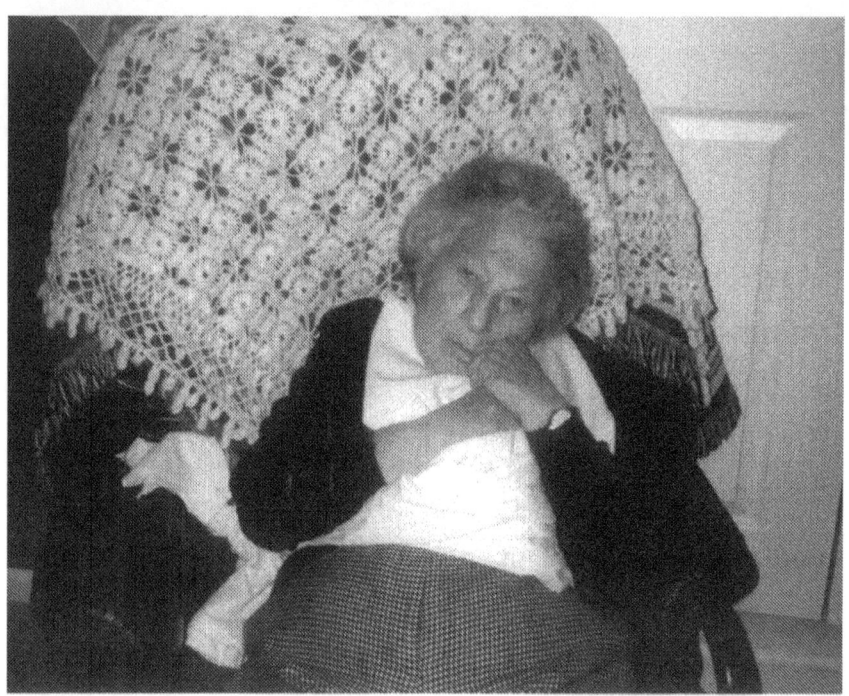

Adele at my home, 2001

*Dementia is a brain disorder that seriously affects a person's ability to carry out daily activities. Alzheimer's disease is the most common form of dementia among older people. It involves the parts of the brain that control thought, memory, and language. Every day scientists learn more, but right now the causes of Alzheimer's disease are still unknown, and there is no cure.

Stage VI

The first part of 2002 was pretty much uneventful. Our routine continues with shopping, doctors, laundry, and awaiting warmer weather. For her 91st birthday in May, we again traveled to Indiana. She loves to ride in the car. We spent her birthday with my children. I got her a cake as usual. Adele's physical health seems to be good but the Alzheimer's has its hold on her. She is not doing well with eating even the pureed food. It is sad to watch her go down but I continue taking her on outings. She talks very little. I say: "Good-night, Adele". She answers: "Good-night". I am grateful for small things as I'm sure she is also, even if she cannot talk.

In July I took Adele to the hairdresser for a perm. I was informed by the hair dresser who knew her family that Marty had died of the Lou Gehrig's disease, just the night before. I was shocked that no one had informed me but after the recent death of Allene, the family must have been devastated.

Adele and I attended the funeral services although Adele was totally unaware of the situation.

One of Marty's sons took over Adele's financial affairs. We saw nothing of her family for quiet some time. Marty's secretary keeps in touch regarding the condition of Adele.

I remembered feeling sad for Adele. Her family was dying off and she was really alone except for my care. I knew then that I would never stop caring for her no matter what happened next. I prayed to God for the strength and health to continue my promise to her. I made that promise in 1997 and I would keep my commitment with the Lord's help.

The year ended again to find Adele and I alone for the Holidays. We are inseparable companions. She has become like my child and I continue to read to her blank expression.

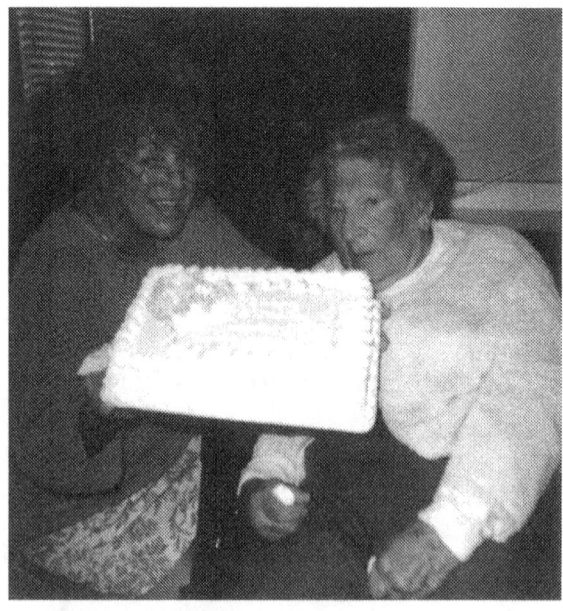

Adele's 91st Birthday

Stage VII

The 2003 winter was long but we still got out. We attended church where a ramp made pushing the wheelchair easier. I pray unceasingly for strength and wisdom to care for Adele.

In May we made our yearly trip to Indiana to visit and have Adele's birthday party. Adele's birthday this year will see her turn 92. I wonder what is God's plan for her and I.

In August the North East has a black out. Adele and I were in the mall on August 14th. We had just left because Adele had an appointment to get her hair cut.

We got into the car and were driving along when I got cut off on my cell phone while talking to my daughter. Next, the traffic lights all went out. When we got to the senior home we were unable to get to her apartment because the elevators were not working.

I got into my car and headed for my home with Adele. I had a generator. My son hooked it up for me and we were able to have lights during the whole black out. The senior home was without power for two days!

Adele and I spent much of this year at my home while repairs were being done. We spent more time at my home and less at the senior complex as days passed.

In late September of this year we drove to Washington D.C. for a family wedding. My family knew that I would not entrust Adele with anyone so they just expected that she would be with me.

This year ended uneventful with the two of us alone again for the Holidays. I wonder sometime, who is caring for whom. My care of Adele is my life. I never think of life without her.

I read to her but I have no way of knowing for sure what she does and does not understand.

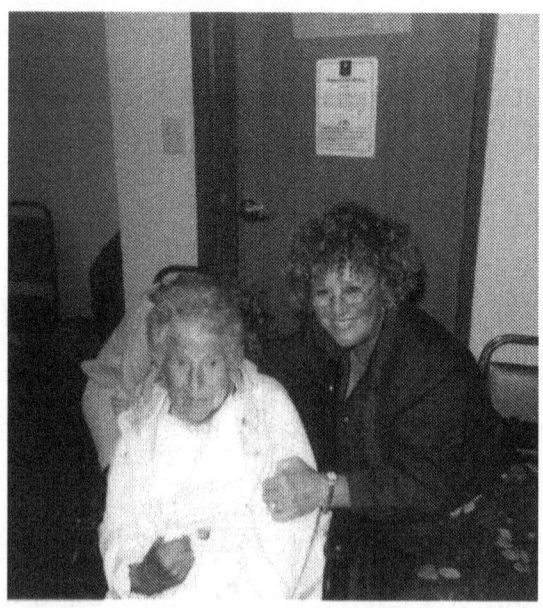

2003 Indiana visit and Birthday celebration

Stage VIII

2004 is the year of ear infections! I carried Adele to the emergency room several times because of these infections. Doctors would prescribe antibiotics to clear these infections only to have them flair up again. Every two months for the entire year, her ears were cleaned out by the doctor but the infections persisted.

In the spring, we traveled to Indiana to visit and celebrate Adele's 93rd birthday. Again, we had a wonderful visit with my children and they also helped to brighten Adele's birthday celebration. She has grown a year older, lost a few pounds, but for the most part she is well and in good health.

Early in the year, on the news, I heard that former President Ronald Regan suffered from Alzheimer's disease. He had been born on February 6, 1911. I noted that Adele had been born May 30, 1911. They shared the same birth year and the same disease. He died on June 5th of this year but Adele lived on. It made me wonder how long she would go on.

For Thanksgiving, we traveled to be with my family at my daughter's home in Indiana. We decided to go back for a visit at Christmas. Adele was happier, it seemed, when we were traveling along. She loves to ride. We arrived back home before the New Year, awaiting the start of 2005.

Stage IX to Present

Adele and I started out 2005 with a mid winter trip in February to visit with my children in Indiana. We spent a seemingly fast week, had fun and returned home.

Upon our return I received a phone call from Adele's nephew, who is in charge of Adele's financial affairs. He was very concerned about the amount of money going out each month for Adele's apartment at the senior home. It was an expense that was cutting deeply into her finances. I thus suggested that we move Adele into my home to cut this expense. After some thought, the nephew agreed to this idea.

I spent the month of March preparing a room in my home for Adele to live in. In April of 2005 Adele moved into my home. Her hospital bed and her belongings made the change minimal for her.

It became a much better situation for both of us. I no longer had to travel from my home to her apartment or worry about my home being empty while I was with Adele.

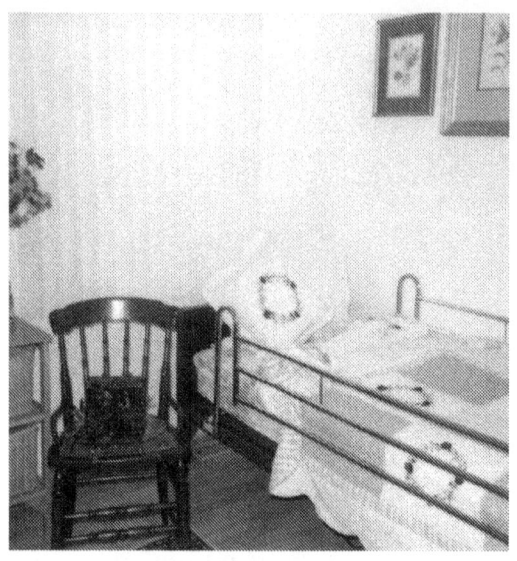

Adele's room in my home

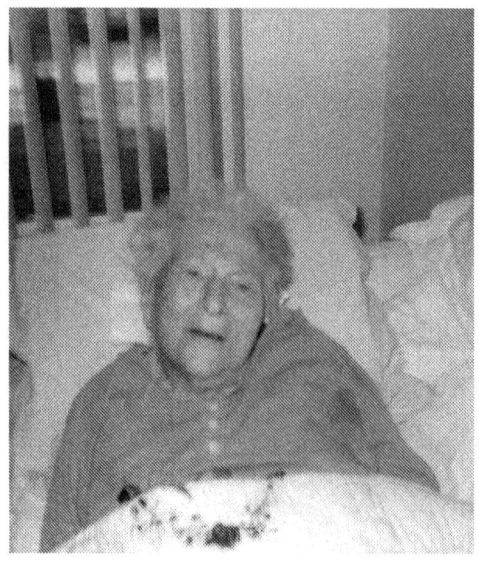

Adele resting in her new home

We discovered that Adele's ear infections might have been caused by a fungus infection contracted through living at the senior home. She no longer had the ear problems after moving into my home. I was so thankful because I could just imagine the pain my dear Adele was going through without being able to voice it. I felt it a blessing she no longer had to suffer.

This year we celebrated Adele's 94th birthday at home. It had taken to much out of me preparing my home for Adele for us to make our usual trip to Indiana. We thus, had a quite celebration.

This stage in our lives continues into 2006 and I care for my little Adele with the same love that made me promise to do so in 1997. I continue to ask God for the grace, strength, and good health needed to continue my labor of love towards His precious child, Adele.

Monday, July 10, 2006

MONDAY, July 10 (HealthDay News) -- Measuring levels of a protein in the cerebrospinal fluid of middle-aged adults at high genetic risk for Alzheimer's disease may reveal early signs of disease development, U.S. researchers report.

A team from the University of Washington, Seattle, noted that aging, plus the presence of a copy of a gene called apolipoprotein E*4 (APOE*4) are the two strongest known risk factors for Alzheimer's. People with APOE*4 develop clinical dementia about 10 to 15 years earlier than people without this particular allele (copy).

Previous research had found that Alzheimer's-related plaques in the brain begin forming years before a person shows any symptoms of the disease. These plaques are made of proteins called beta-amyloids, predominately a type known as "A beta 42." As these proteins clump together into plaques, there are fewer circulating through the nervous system.

According to the researchers, this means that lower levels of A beta 42 in the cerebrospinal fluid surrounding the brain and spinal cord are an indicator of the development of Alzheimer's disease.

The study, published in the July *Archives of Neurology*, included 184 adults, average age 50 years, who had no symptoms of Alzheimer's disease. Researchers checked each participant for the APOE*4 allele and took samples of cerebrospinal fluid to check their levels of A beta 42.

People who were older and had the APOE*4 allele were more likely to have lower levels of A beta 42 than people without the APOE*4 allele. The researchers concluded that people with the APOE*4 allele experienced a slight decline in A beta 42 in their younger years and then a dramatic decline between 50 and 60 years old.

Those without the APOE*4 allele have a slight increase in A beta 42 levels until age 50, and then experience a gradual decline in those levels.

"In persons with the APOE*4 allele, decline in cerebrospinal fluid A beta 42 concentration possibly begins in young adulthood, followed by marked acceleration of this decline beginning in midlife-decades before clinical manifestation of Alzheimer's disease," the study authors wrote.

"These findings have implications for the preclinical diagnosis of Alzheimer's disease, as well as for treatment," they added. "Therapeutic strategies aimed at prevention of Alzheimer's disease may need to be applied in early midlife or even younger ages to have maximal effect on amyloid deposition. Primary prevention trials for Alzheimer's disease targeting elderly persons may [already] be too late to affect the early stages of disease pathology."

Its now 2006 and the year starts out well. Adele is doing as well as can be expected. She will be 95 this May 30th. Feeding Adele is getting more difficult as she would clamp her teeth togeather and it was getting almost impossible to hand feed her. I went to a nearby pharmacy that sold a large tube syringe with a nozzle for sucking. This device turned out to be great for feeding. I am still using it to this day to get nourishment into my friend Adele and she is doing great.

We took our usual trip to see my children in Indiana and had a small birthday party for Adele's 95th.

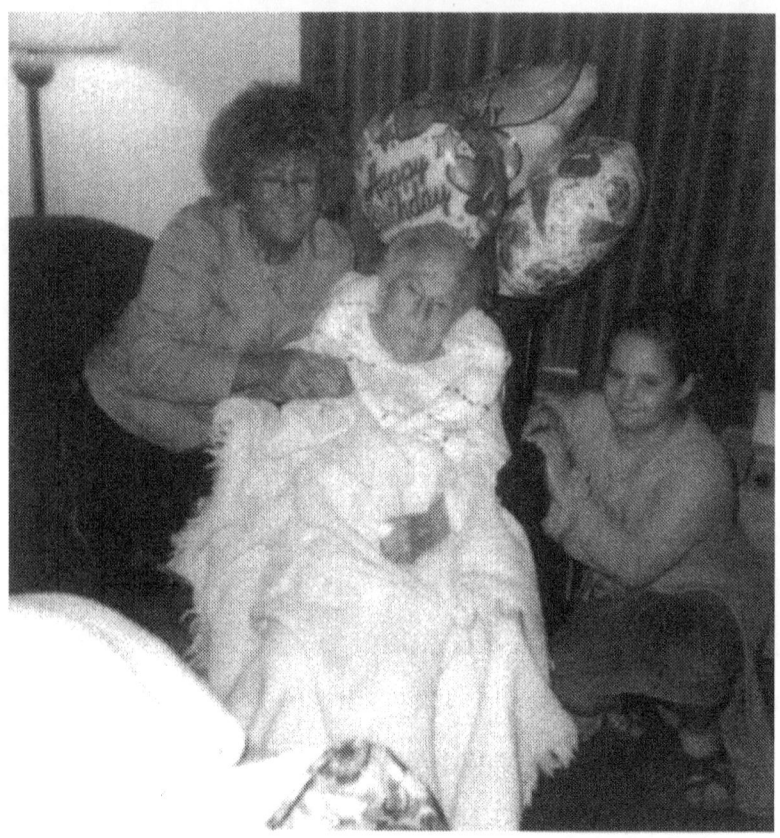

Adele's 95th Birthday Party with my granddaughter

I continue to take Adele to the beauty parlor regularly to get her haircut and a perm, although less frequently than in earlier years. This latest appointment was in July and it is pictured here. I also have included one of Adele's many visits to Dr. Eisenberg's office pictuerd with nurse Jody.

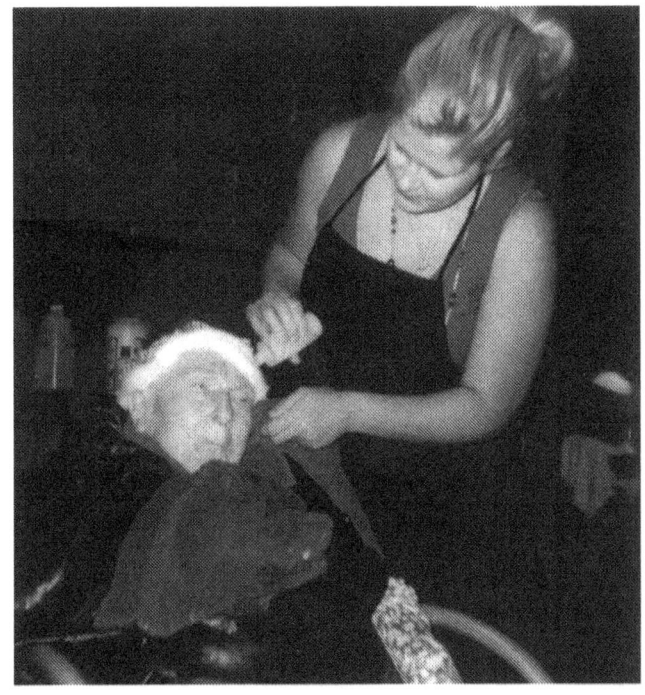

Adele getting hair cut and perm

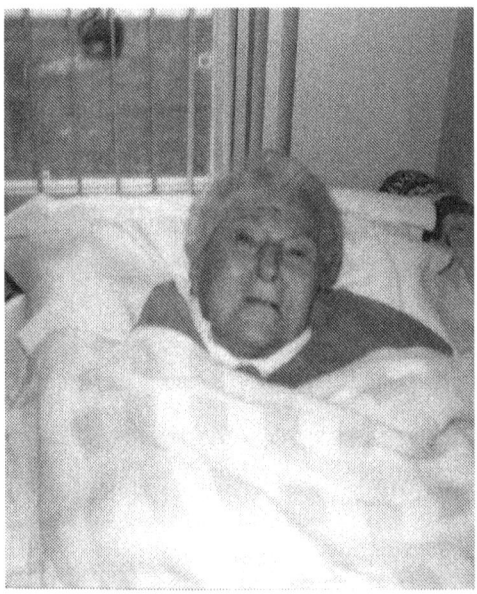

Adele back home after hair cut and perm

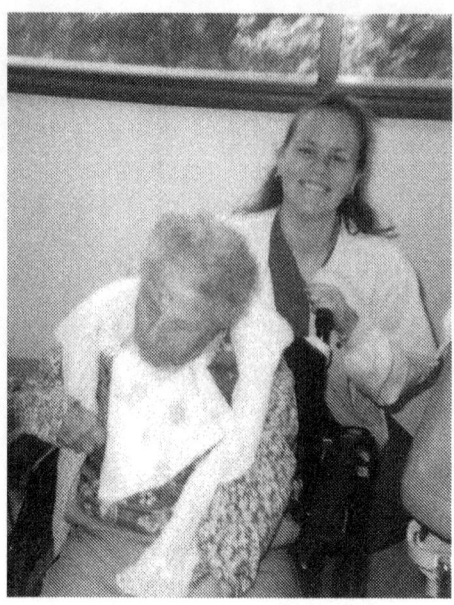

Adele at one of many doctors visits

In August of this year, I got a distressful phone call from the great nephew who is handling Adele's funds. He told me that he will make arrangements very soon to put Adele into a nursing home. Her funds for care are almost gone. This was not a happy day for me, as I knew money was getting low. I was praying that I would have time to publish this book to have money to keep caring for Adele in my home. I continue to pray that this can still happen. I close this chapter with a prayer of faith that the Lord will take care of it all. Faith and peace to all who find comfort from this story.

The year 2007 brings us to the final chapter of this saga. January 11, ushered in a very heart breaking day. Adele's great nephew came to visit, and had decided it was time to put his great aunt into a nursing home before all of her funds were depleted. His reasoning was, by placing her in a nursing home prior to her funds running out, she could be placed in a more up scale environment. This would prevent her from going into a less desirable environment because of a lack of adequete funds in the future.

For the next 13 days, x-ray technicians and various doctors came to evaluate Adeles condition and assess the required care, which would enable her to be placed in the most accommodating nursing home. All arrangments had been completed, and on January 24th at 10am the nursing home transportation vehicle arrived to take away my little friend. Needless to say, this was one of the worst days I have ever experienced in my entire life. I spent the remainder of the day crying and reminiscing after having her in my care for the past 10 years. It was very hard to let my little friend go.

The following day I received a call from a nurse at the nursing home inquiring as to what Adele normally ate. After informing her of my normal routine when it came to feeding Adele, the nurse told me Adele would not take any food without choking. This made me very sad because I had fed her prior to her leaving, and there was no problem with her feeding. She had consumed her normal feeding of 2 cups of ensure, water, liquid iron, and flax seed oil without any choking problems. However, I did not give her any baby food or juice upon her departure, because I felt it may have been to much for her to handle along with the ride.

On Friday, I received a call from the nephew's wife stating, she was proceeding to get a court order which would prevent Adele from getting a feeding tube inserted into her stomach for feeding. Initially, I agreed with this, for I did not want Adele to suffer from this procedure. However, what I was to soon discover the following day upon my visit to the nursing home to see my dear friend, is that the court order also prevented Adele from receiving any water.

After I arrived at the nursing home the nurse told me that she would not eat and when I attempted to give her some water, the nurse told me the only thing I could do would be to swab her lips with a damp cotton swab. I made a second attempt to give my friend some water; however, again I was told by the nurse it was forbidden by law to give her any water. At that, I just held my little friend of 10 years in my arms, kissed her, told her I loved her and said my final goodbye. I left the visit with my little friend very upset, as her eyes looked so frighten that it just broke my heart knowing how she was to die. I could not return for another visit, seeing her suffering and knowing what was going to happen in the next few days, was just to much for me to bear.

I would call the nephews home for an update on Adele's condition. I spoke with the nephew's wife after her visit on February 1st, and was told they had placed a morphine patch on Adele for pain. Realizing the pain she must have been suffering, just upset me that much more. Two days later, Saturday, February 3rd, I called the nursing home to inquire about the condition of Adele, and was told I would have to contact the family for any further information, they were not allowed to speak to me regarding her condition. Thus, I called the nephew and got the answering machine, so I left a message asking them to give me a call regarding Adele's condition. During this waiting period, I can't help but think, she has passed away.

The following day, Sunday, I went to the early church services and hoped I would receive a call from the nephew upon my return home. The call did come, and I was told that my little friend, Adele, had passed away early that morning. I cryed a lot that day. Even though I new it was inevitable, I couldn't hold back the tears. The pain I felt with the loss of my little Adele was almost unbearable. I called on God much this day to ease my pain and I prayed he would grant a home for my friend in heaven.

As I continued to cry because of the loss of my dear friend, I began to recall something she mentioned to me some time ago. I mentioned earlier that she had been a school teacher for many years. She told me how she would stress to her students the importance of learning how to make a budget to pay bills and save some of their earnings when they began working. She was an english teacher and such a lady of character, she told me she felt in addition to teaching the structured subject matter, the students needed every day life lessons. She and her husband never had any biological children; however, I can imagine how she mothered the many students she taught throughout her years of teaching. I know, just the couple of years we were together and her mind was still somewhat good, I was able to learn so much from her. She has touched my life like no other person has.

I also recall her telling me her mother had Alzheimers and that she and her sister Jenny both paid for her nursing home care. Adele and I talked a lot in the first year or so, in my job as her caregiver.

Thinking back when I first started with Adele, I had a dog named Chico, who at the time was 18 years old and not in the best of health. Because of the time I was now spending with Adele, it had become almost impossible for me to care for my dog as he needed. Thus, I concluded, the best thing for Chico was to have him put to sleep. On the day I asked a friend to take him to the vet to take care of this matter, I mentioned to Adele how this was not a happy day for me because of the situation with my dog. She suggested that we go to a restaurant for lunch to get my mind off of Chico. However, while sitting in the restaurant, I could not eat, knowing Chico would not be at home when I returned and I began to cry. While I'm sitting and crying over the loss of my dog of 18 years, Adele suddenly asked, " I wonder who will cry when I die". In my recalling this incident 10 years later, I guess it was me.

On the day I learned of Adele's passing, I took a copy of the picture on the front of this book and a rose to the senior home where she had lived for 10 years to place on the counter for those who may have known her, would know she had passed on.

On Tuesday February 6th, there was a grave side service for my dear friend, Adele. There were only about 12 people present, consisting primaryly of great neices and newphews, for she had out lived all other family members. I placed a ½ dozen pink roses on her grave. As I stood there before her little coffin crying my eyes out, I kept thinking how much she had enriched my life over the past 10 years, and how much I would miss her in my life. Although, over the latter years it became increasingly harder to care for her, I will miss all of that.

I have learned so much from my little friend Adele, who I will always miss. I am sure she is looking down from the balcony of heaven as I write these words.

"I love you Adele".

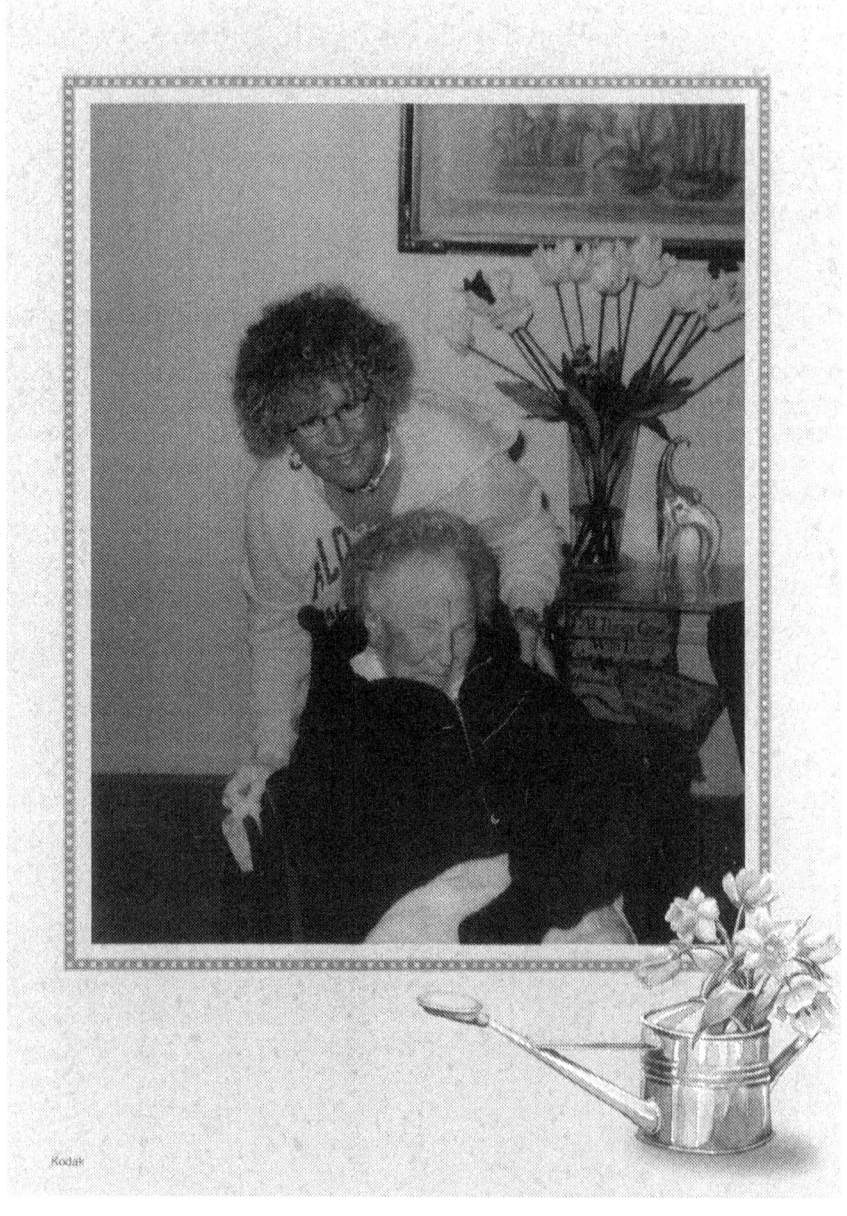

Adele just before trip to nursing home